Thunderclap

The Doctor and the Brain Bleed

Thunderclap

The Doctor and the Brain Bleed

AMIT BHARKHADA

CONTENTS

DEDICATION

In Indian mythology, the Tree of Life is known as the *Akshaya Vata* or *Immortal Tree*. If one branch is struck, the rest of the tree channels its own resources to the damaged part to help it heal and grow.

For:

Rasik and Mahisha

My parents. For providing and cultivating strong roots, deeply planted in a rich earth of sound values, boundless love and constant nurturing. *"A tree with strong roots laughs at storms"* - *Malay proverb*

Viren and Anisha

My brother and sister-in-law: fellow branches of the tree of life, lending me their strength to heal and grow back when I was struck.

Rian and Siya

My wondrous children, for being the magical fruits of life.

Nilesh and Bharti

Sona's parents, for helping with the healing and recovery. And for creating ...

Sona

My darling wife. When we are together, I become whole again and the tree blossoms. Home is wherever you are.

ABOUT THE AUTHOR

Amit Bharkhada is ...

An experienced GP Principal at Jubilee Medical Practice in Syston, Leicestershire.

Passionate about research and has presented at international conferences in Japan, The Netherlands, Scotland and UK national events.

Clinical Director of Strategy at LLR Training Hub: particularly interested in workforce development and transformation through the education and training of Healthcare Professionals.

Honorary Associate Professor at De Montfort University, Faculty of Health and Life Sciences.

Holder of the PGCert in Medical Education and Member of the Academy of Medical Educators and Royal College of General Practitioners.

A son who loves his parents
A husband who loves his wife
A father who loves his children
A brother who loves his brother and family
A friend to friends

And, most recently, a patient who experienced and is recovering from a sub-arachnoid haemorrhage. (A particularly nasty brain bleed, for non-medical readers.)

And that - the last and least welcome addition to this list of who I am - is what this book is about: the before, the during and the after of an event that changes you in ways both profound and subtle, including how you see your own life and the people around you.

I learnt a lot crossing the wall from doctor to patient.
I'm sharing that in these pages.

CHAPTER 1. BANG! OUT OF THE BLUE

"Time is the most valuable thing a man can spend" -
Theophrastus

Out of the blue, or, even more unexpectedly, from inside yourself, comes a sudden 'event' - such a small word for when this thing strikes - that knocks you off the path of normal life, where the future - the next second, minute, hour, morning, afternoon, evening, day, week, month, years - have a predictable pattern to them; in which you are moving on and up through an infinite series of tiny, momentary presents, with the actions in each present forming a future of growing, learning, contributing and enjoying, ageing, slowly changing into the person and the life you will lead; the delight of watching your children grow, the professional challenges ahead, the career progression that hard work should bring, because it always has done.

All that future, much of it conscious, much of it an unconscious stream in which you feel you are flowing with an unspoken sense of inevitability, is suspended suddenly by an event in the present that pulls the ground from under you, threatens to sweep away all of that future life. It's a moment that changes everything and suspends all possible futures.

The medics call it a thunderclap moment. You change, morph from doctor to patient, from unquestionably alive to at risk of not being, from juggling all the balls we are dealt with in life: home, work, kids, spouse, parents, sibling, colleagues, patients, friends - the net of relationships through which we live our lives, express ourselves, serve, love, grow and learn - all of that is suspended, frozen in time suddenly by this thing inside that taps you, agonisingly, on the inside of your head - as if that head is no longer yours - and says:

"All that - everything you knew as your life - is suspended for now. You need to pay attention to me. Because I've taken you to the edge. And forced you to look over at what might be. And then look back again at that web of life, of people you love and serve, and see them, and yourself, differently. One way or the other, you'll never be the same again."

Like so many life-changing days, it didn't look that way from the start. It was just another ordinary day.

Wednesday 9th August 2023 – a normal day in the life of a busy GP surgery.

We talk of 'work-life balance' as if one is discrete from the other. This is, of course, a nonsense, a false dichotomy. Work is wrapped into your life for a large part of each day. So, in terms of probability (work out how many hours in any given twenty-four your life experience is set in the workplace, to give you the percentage probability), some of your biggest life events will inevitably be experienced at work.

Midweek is a fulcrum in the timeline of the mind. You look back at what you've achieved so far. You look forward to your commitments for the rest of the week. It's an unconscious assessment point, a liminal place, balanced halfway between immediate past and immediate future.

This day would be more than that for me; a turning point of sorts in my life, or at least an inflection point after which the way I saw my life would change forever.

It started, as usual, with the intense focus of a full clinical morning. Some mornings are face to face clinical appointments. This morning was a telephone clinic.

Then came a teaching session with the Postgraduate Doctors in Training (PGDiT in the jargon). I love teaching as much as doctoring.

Then came a Microsoft Teams meeting.

All normal so far, I think you'll agree. Obviously, your sense of aliveness and fulfilment, of usefulness and enjoyment of life in the moments that make up a morning move up and down through a normal midweek morning such as this. Not that you are that aware of the real-time graph of your life experiences, the highs and lows, as it rises and falls in the moment, like micro-movements in the stock market, in an ordinary day. Our sense of our inner workings - of how we feel - doesn't tend to be a preoccupation, in the moment. You're a doctor. You're there for your patients, colleagues, and trainees. You are outwardly focused; you are on duty. That duty is to others. You're there to serve.

Yes, even if the medium through which you are serving is a Microsoft Teams meeting.

Which finished at 1pm.

My last normal morning for the near future was over. That 1pm was the last normal minute of my life, in fact. No, let's not exaggerate. There were five more normal, usual, mundane minutes of that former life, the me that was before the Thunderclap moment.

Which happened at 1.05pm.

I felt a sudden 'Thunderclap!' at the back of my head. 'Out of the blue,' we say, don't we, as if these unexpecteds are visited upon us from outside, thrown at us from the blue sky above. We don't expect our autonomously working, healthy inside to suddenly, treacherously you might say if you were feeling dramatic, strike a blow from within - the system that sustains us and **is** us turning on us Unthinkable. Threats come from outside, don't they? That's where threat and danger live.

That kind of melodramatic thinking didn't go through my head.

I was out of sync with what was happening within.

For me, this was still a normal day.

A normal day with a sudden headache.

What went through my head (in fact, in response to the pain of the abnormal event, a pain which was also going through my head, of course) was the rational doctor processes medics are trained in:

"Tell me more about the pain," we are trained to say sympathetically to patients when they report a pain to us, aren't we?

Working through the clinical diagnostic reasoning process, my doctor's head answered my doctor's question as I automatically went through the headache algorithm:

Where is the pain; when did it start; how would you characterise it; what makes it better or worse; does it radiate; what's the severity score; are there other symptoms?

And so on to try and deduce the diagnosis and causation. My right shoulder didn't quite feel right. It felt ... odd. So, what's the diagnosis?

My doctor colleague was working in the opposite room and he had his door open. He noticed I was in pain and offered me paracetamol, which I took. But I then started to develop neck pain and noticed the light was irritating my eyes - I was photosensitive. I lay on the patient examining couch to see if that would help.

Our actions, I discovered in these moments, are a form of feedback that tell us something is not right, as if we are observing someone else doing these odd things, have stepped outside the normal course of what was supposed to happen next, and are acting, well, weirdly. A bit of you thinks, "What on earth are you doing? This isn't how these next few moments were supposed to be."

It was dawning on me that this - whatever I was experiencing - seemed something more serious than a run-of-the-mill headache.

It's in these moments that we realise we maintain several different realities in our heads. The one mainstream 'normal' reality is dominant - the predictable one that you had planned for the day and where you know what comes next. Other possibilities merely lurk far beneath as unlikely undercurrents that are not even part of your aware mind. When these unwelcome alternative realities start to well up into your consciousness, summoned there to explain the abnormal sensations your body is feeding to you, the natural reaction is to downplay them in your mind. They start to sit there, an unwelcome addition to the normal reality, now alongside instead of buried beneath, but you don't let them (not yet anyway) oust your normal reality as the most likely one you are experiencing.

You damp it down. Crossing that line from doctor to patient, even in your head? That's not a line you cross willingly.

About ten minutes later two nurse colleagues popped in for a quick chat. They instantly saw I didn't look right. I guess the lights being out and the doctor prone on the patient couch rather than smiling at them from behind his desk were clues.

The surprise at this unexpected scene was momentary as my colleagues shifted quickly to professional mode. You see it happen when there's an accident in the street, when someone goes down. The ones who spontaneously run towards it are the medics, the nurses. It just kicks in. It's instinct. It's who you are.

They asked rather urgently how I was.

When I explained my symptoms, one of them asked absolutely the right and only question to ask a doctor in that moment:

"What would you do if this was a patient?"

The question helped me over that line I was so reluctant to step over.

"Admit", said a voice. It was my voice.

"Right, you are going in. I'm driving you", one of them said.

I was reluctant. We always are when we have to tug ourselves out of the habitual, preferred normal stream of life, aren't we - all the things people were relying on me to do that afternoon were flying through my head! - and tread onto what may be a more dangerous path.

Denial is such a powerful thing.

But my medical training told me that I had to do this. Reluctantly, I agreed it was probably the safest option. But, I didn't want to take yet more colleagues out of the surgery as well as myself.

"My wife will take me", I said.

Nottingham, I knew, was the nearest neurosurgical centre. This is where working in the medical profession means that you have insight into where might be best to go when something odd is happening to you.

I called Sona, my wife.

Sona is a director of Radfield Home Care, Leicester, and she had a meeting locally that lunchtime. When I called, she was walking back to the office (just 5 minutes from my work).

I said, "You need to take me to hospital. I have an atypical headache - it's quite bad."

I sensed the surprise in her voice as she said, "I am a few minutes away. I am coming."

She turned around and headed my way. The words were transactional, with both of us prioritising getting to the hospital over-sharing how we felt. But we were so close that we each had a sense of the underlying concerns of the other. I met her at my car in the surgery car park and she drove us towards Nottingham.

There was a strange, tense feeling in the car during that drive. Being in the presence of your soulmate, the person you are most at ease with in life, the person who is most an extension of you and vice versa, yet being unsure what to say, is the strangest sensation. The combination of the familiar (driving in the car together with my wife) with the unfamiliar (that we were heading into the unknown) was surreal. We chatted. But the subject matter felt alien as it came out of our mouths.

"This could be something serious," I said at one point, followed quickly by, "Lucky we have a will." ('Lucky' – interesting choice of words as we try to see the positive). I always say to people that once you have children, make sure you get a will made. Throwing that in after "This could be serious" was like offering a cushion to provide a soft landing, I guess, almost to ameliorate the preceding statement. A rather inadequate cushion, of course; you grab at whatever you can in these circumstances.

But then we both spotted what had been missed out. Neither of us had drawn up a medical Lasting Power of Attorney (LPA). There are two types of LPA for when a person's ability to make or communicate decisions about what they want to happen next is compromised. The better-known is Power of Attorney for property and financial affairs – who makes decisions about your money and property. The less well-known – and less well-practised in terms of being enacted ready for when the worst might happen – is an LPA stating who makes decisions about you, about your health and welfare, if you can't.

We prepare more for what to do with what we own when we become incapable of voicing decisions than what to do with who we are. This was the first emergence of a questioning watchfulness as if observing my own situation and tracking back to how we arrived here. Were we prepared? I was oddly pleased – you look for anything that shows you did in fact prepare for this unknown territory you find yourself in – that I'd made a will, as not many people of my age have, and that preparation implies a kind of prescience, that life hasn't spun completely out of control, that you had accounted for and covered this possible future.

Followed by the minor deflation of having missed the medical LPA. Sona picked up on it because, she said – and this is the odd synchronicity that you notice at times when life seems to be spinning out of control, as you look for meaning to hang onto – that she and her colleagues had been discussing LPAs just a couple of hours ago, before the call came through from me. When we discuss these things as they apply to patients and others it doesn't occur to us that – as in Sona's case – she will get a call shortly after in which the absence of an LPA becomes glaringly obvious in our own lives.

The self-questioning races through you at times like this: "Have we had the right conversations in life? No LPA! So, God forbid if I lost capacity." Who would be the decision makers? Without an LPA it wouldn't legally or automatically be Sona, the person who knows me best and whom I would want to entrust with intuiting what I want in any given situation if I can't comprehend or articulate it for myself.

So, clear learning here: If you do not have a medical LPA, look into it: you want to plan ahead for health eventualities that you may not want to think or talk about – organisations practise 'disaster planning' after all, but families and individuals don't usually, as there are futures we would rather not imagine or upset our loved ones by raising.

These thoughts were racing through both our heads when we arrived at the hospital A&E, Sona dropping me off as she went to find a parking space. Walking through those doors as a patient rather than a doctor felt odd to say the least. I couldn't quite believe it.

While Sona was parking, my brain – injured though it had been by something - was continuing to whir away to try and work out what the 'thing' that had attacked it was and what might happen next. A doctor's brain, when under attack, becomes the ultimate self-diagnosing machine, I'd discovered. Shame that couldn't extend to self-healing.

The potential nature of the event in my head that had brought me here, through the doors of A&E, was the problem to be solved as Sona walked in from the car park, sat and held my hand. "How serious could this be?" was the obvious preoccupation, followed immediately by the long train of unwelcome consequences: "What is the impact this will have on my family, my children, Sona?" We are normally in control of the impact we have on the lives of those we love. The thought that your own and their wellbeing is out of your hands and that something that is happening inside you could hurt – massively – both yourself and them is the most unwelcome and unanticipated state of mind - and being -you can find yourself in.

The rationalising - rapid processing of possible future outcomes, weighing up of probabilities - continued during the time spent in A&E as, like everyone else in there, we waited 'patiently' for our turn. The doctor's natural inclination and training is to have your attention turned outwards on patients, to observe and analyse them rather than yourself. Surrounded by patients, I found my mind returning to this programming. I remember registering so many different emotions in the people around me.

You could see sadness in the face of one, pain, bewilderment, quiet resignation in others. There was the relief apparent in those who were being discharged, heading for that exit door back out into a world where they themselves decided what would happen next, as rapidly as they could, keen to escape it seemed in one or two cases, just in case someone changed their minds and called them back for another long wait. What is our most powerful need beyond the basics of life? To be in control of what comes next, to lead our own lives.

All human life was there, as they say, in different states of need and distress, some more obvious than others. The medic in me noticed the limping people, the lady with a cut thumb and significant bleeding. There were tableaux of distress: A woman who appeared to be intoxicated was shouting angrily, surrounded by security guards. But, also tableaux of tenderness and care: An elderly gentleman who looked to be in his 90s was being pushed in a wheelchair by another elderly gentlemen. A partially-sighted patient was there with a guide dog. The twitch, the urge to do something for these people, had to be held in check by the constant mental reminder that I was here as a patient, as were they.

During the hours we were there, I saw so much to admire in the work of the A&E staff, but inevitably felt for the patients having to wait so long. A theme that permeates this book was seeded here, in this A&E waiting room: there are limits to how much understanding a doctor's empathy can provide about a patient's position. Being there, in the other person's shoes, isn't something you would want to do. But being for an extended length of time in the patient's position, observing, feeling, sharing the patient experience from their side of it, brings with it invaluable learning. That is one of my motivations, of course – encapsulating and sharing that learning – in writing this little book.

As time went on in A&E, another part of my brain – the part causing the pain - drew my attention from the people and the environment around me back to what was going on inside: the pain was increasing. And a stiffness in my neck had become more pronounced. Could this be a sub-arachnoid haemorrhage (SAH)? The more the clock ticked past, the more symptoms appeared, the more the odds seemed to be stacking up against me.

The pain was unreal. Around 6pm, I asked for Paracetamol. It didn't come. One of the consequences of that level of demand in A&E, I thought to myself, and I didn't make a fuss or repeat the request. It is what it is. You could be 'clinical' about it and say, as some analyses have, that some of the demand in that room was overspill from the pressure on primary care; that people were coming in inappropriately and putting up with the wait to make sure they were seen by a doctor at some point. I looked around. If anyone was being looked at with a "Why are you here? Is it really necessary?" eye, it would be me, wouldn't it. No limp or visible injury or open distress, no blood or bandages or moaning.

The day moved to evening, the clock continued to tick, people in various states of unwellness continued to file, shuffle or be wheeled in and, in various apparent states of relief or continued distress, were allowed out again. I hadn't had any lunch, in fact hadn't even drunk any water at work in the morning, just powered through as we all so often do, don't we, postponing what our body needs in favour of the tasks and responsibilities we are ploughing through. As the hours passed and Sona offered to get me something to eat, I demurred, with the thought that a 'nil by mouth' surgical procedure was one of the possible outcomes branching into the near future in my head. But, by 7pm, I simply had to eat. The ebb and flow continued all around us. It was about 9 pm when the A&E doctor got to me. I asked if it was ok for Sona to join us. He said, "Of course - if that's what you would like." They took us into the consultation bay and we sat. He listened carefully to my brief history and arranged for a CT head scan, which was exactly appropriate and expected, of course. Taking a look inside was the only thing that would really tell us what was going on in there. Sona and I returned to the waiting area.

As the evening wore on, a familiar and welcome figure walked in through the A&E doors; my brother Viren, himself a medic, came to take over from Sona. The children had been picked up from school and were at home with my parents.

Sona needed to get back to them. Viren was reassuring, calming and in his usual way inquisitively thorough in making sure the right steps were being taken. Two fraternal medical heads are better than one. Especially when one of those heads is apparently under attack from the inside.

I was sent for the CT head scan, then we went back to wait the results out. The A&E doctor called us and said the scan was normal. At last, good news! A gap in the clouds appears. Maybe there is nothing to worry about after all. Time to dismantle the worry and possible worst outcomes that had built up in the head and heart over the previous hours? Apparently not. Before elation could set in and displace the worry, there was a 'but'. And it was a big but.

It had been more than six hours between the symptoms presenting themselves – the Thunderclap headache – and the scan. The guidelines, said the A&E doctor, were that we should get a lumbar puncture done to rule out the possibility of a SAH that was lingering in all our heads (possibly literally in mine). Of course, part of me wanted to bolt for the outside world now, as that's where normal life was, last time I was there. The lumbar puncture involved a needle being inserted in the lower back to extract some of the cerebral spinal fluid (CSF) to see if there was anything in there that shouldn't be – something that would confirm an SAH had taken place.

"Really?" I thought. "Is that really necessary?" Of course it was, but this was the remnant of the me that thirty seconds before had been told the scan was clear and was ready to walk out the door, a door which was being closed in my face. I had to push at it a bit. Viren and I negotiated. I asked the doctor what he would do in my position. He turned the answer around slightly and his choice of words made me realise I had to stay:

"For your wife's sake," he said meaningfully, "I would suggest you stay and have the lumbar puncture done tomorrow." Well, that brought it home to me, the seriousness of my situation, and closed the escape route back to normalcy, those images that 'all clear' had opened in my head of Viren taking me home, me hugging the kids and Sona, all of us smiling with relief, life back to normal, at least for now. That wasn't what came next after all. All objections gone. I would be staying the night.

It was about midnight. They'd try and get me a bed, they said, but it might be quite a while. I told Viren to head off home, as this would be a long wait. I had, in the back of my mind, always wondered what it would be like to be on a corridor bed - particularly having worked in A&E before. Placed to one side of a thoroughfare, against a wall, unmoving in a place of movement, everything and everyone else flowing past; the noise, the bustle, while you wait; no place for you, stranded in a place that isn't designed to be a place of rest, of treatment, not even designed to be a waiting place, but an in-between place, somewhere you should be passing through that you end up left in, no place of your own for you here yet. Parked.

So, now I found out. That night I was on a bed, in a corridor, in a row of several other patients, looking oddly as if we were in a queue of some sort. Which in fact we were, of course. I'd worked nights in hospitals, but this was my first overnight stay as a patient, experiencing the hospital night prone on a bed in a corridor. When you are parked, waiting, in a corridor at night, not a lot of sleep happens. The boredom mixes with the anxiety about why you are there, the uncertainty of when someone will appear to move you, the outcome of the planned lumbar puncture (in my case), thoughts of what is happening at home and how they all are, the worry you may be causing them.

Life is defined by change and movement. In death, we are unmoving, outside the stream of life. The irony of leaving our hospital patients unmoving, in a state of limbo in a corridor, in the deep of the night (when time passes most slowly), with the occasional evidence of life passing them in the corridor, is that we are placing them in an unintentional simulacrum of the one end-state of this hospital admissions process that they fear the most. Physically it might be the only safe place they can be, with no beds in wards available. Psychologically, not so much.

When you are on a corridor, your mind strays in the night to those around you, each of the people lined up with me, imagining each of their stories, their issues, their problems, the impact of those on their loved ones, how they might be feeling.

In a corridor, there is no privacy, of course. The emotions of those around you are revealed to you in body language and facial expressions, and you inadvertently study and absorb, reading their experience and, again, learning the limits of empathy. I had been one of the doctors walking past beds in a corridor and empathising with the patients there. But you don't get it until you experience it.

I recall looks of concern passing between patients and their loved ones, hugs, comfort being given, outbursts of anger, all human emotions under stress laid out there in the corridor. The power of non-verbal communication. Part and parcel of the mix of emotions around and within me, and a contributor to them, was the enhanced sense of helplessness that being left in a corridor inevitably brings.

The pain continued. Around 3 a.m., the registrar wrote up Morphine and Paracetamol to take the edge off. The night wore on.

Vulnerability is the de facto state of a patient in hospital, not a state any of us welcomes and one of the staff, in my experience, do everything they can to alleviate in terms of reassurance and confidence that you are in safe hands. But, the underlying truth of the situation, of our status when we become patients, is that being in hospital is beyond our control. Being in the hands of others, being cared for and needing to trust them was something I wasn't used to. When it's normally the other way around, it is strange to be cast on the other side of the drama. Because there is a drama to this – a 'What comes next?' uncertainty has crept into your life story. You are no longer in control.

In the early hours of the morning, I was transferred to the Medical Assessment Unit (MAU). The Consultant visited later that morning and planned to arrange the lumbar puncture. Now, I've done them myself, of course. I was, though, apprehensive. It's a large needle. When the Medical Registrar who was to do mine came to my bedside to fill in my consent form with me, she had a Senior House Officer

(SHO) with her. I couldn't stop myself from asking the obvious question. Which I'll outline in the next section of this book, a section that focuses on the leadership learning I picked up observing my colleagues in action, from the perspective of being on the receiving end and observing, so to speak.

Key points:
1. Consider planning a will, particularly where dependents exist
2. Talk openly with trust when discussing LPA in your home environment
3. The human imperative is to be in control
4. Observations of non-verbal communication should be acknowledged

CHAPTER 2. WHAT THE PATIENT SAW: LEADERSHIP AND COMMUNICATION

"The great sociologist Max Weber said, over 100 years ago, that the organisations that will survive and thrive will be those that foster acts of leadership throughout the system, rather than assuming leadership only exists at the top." - Phil Dourado, leadership development expert

'Acts of leadership throughout the system' is more or less a definition of what the NHS aims for: systems leadership, also known as systemic leadership. The ideal is that every member of every team knows their role (and everybody else's) within the system and how their actions impact on the wider care of the patient, with all parties guided by the imperative of providing integrated, person-centred, co-ordinated care.

Yes, that sounds idealistic. Also, a bit mechanistic? Systems leadership originates in Taichi Ohno's carmaking system at Toyota (where any worker can raise their hand to stop and adjust the process because they feel there is a quality problem, and the bosses listen and act on that). Its theoretical roots lie in the thinking of W. Edwards Deming - the father of Total Quality Management, which Deming himself criticised when it was so often enacted as box-ticking bureaucracy rather than a set of lived values.

But, don't let that put you off. At its best, what we get from NHS healthcare practitioners who practise systemic leadership is indeed organic in look and feel. I've watched and been part of teams where the inter and intra teamwork is, yes, systemic in its scope, but in the sense of a living system - symbiotic, almost intuitive, like a single organism working to the same end, with the same set of values, purpose and desired outcomes; a self-improving system made up of self-improving individuals and teams, learning from practice and each other as we go, working within a clear framework and set of processes guided by a common vision and values. Leadership and direction are embedded in the system, within the practitioners and their interaction with each other and the patient, as Weber predicted an ideal state should be.

Brilliant NHS teams, when delivering to the patient, can look like mind-readers, all seeming to follow the same invisible script in a seamless delivery of care wrapped around the patient. There is a sense of a hive mind, almost, with the NHS at its best.

Yes, of course, that's an ideal. Yes, of course, demand growth and restricted resources strain the ideal we aim for, at times to breaking point. But, what I want to report here is that my experience revealed excellence of practice in teamwork and distributed leadership that inspired trust in me, the patient. I was in quiet awe of some of what I saw and experienced. You may never have seen these practices from the patient's perspective. I've shared some of what I learnt from the A&E and night-in-the-corridor experience earlier in this book. This chapter and the next dig deeper into learning from the patient experience - ***this*** patient's experience.

So, we start with the lumbar puncture that, in the last chapter, we left patient Amit discussing with the Registrar at his bedside:

"Are you doing it?" I asked, eyeing the SHO accompanying her.

We all know how it works in doctoring, how we learn new procedures: Halsted's Model, which originated in 1890, is always shorthanded to;

See one
Do one
Teach one

When put as baldly as that, it sounds alarming. I'd never thought about that before - how internal shorthand can, if known by the patient and taken literally, be scary. No-one wants to be practised on. But of course, that's exactly who I was at that point: the patient. Hence the insight. Which I share here. It's so valuable to have that perspective for when I'm back on the doctor side of the doctor/patient roles.

The six words are an abbreviation of process, not a literal description of actuality. Though it was taken literally in 1890 - a *stretch target* to use modern jargon - when it was seen as an actual description of cascaded learning, raising the expectation that if you hadn't learnt a new procedure through one observation, you weren't performing to expectation. We are more concerned with patient safety and practitioner accountability now, to be that literal, thank goodness. There's supervision, there's increasing levels of independence until the trainee is judged able to do it themselves. There's more than 'one' in other words, for each of those three steps. Yet we still use the shorthand. Maybe even find it edgy and a bit thrilling? The nuance and meaning of all our language, our jargon and shorthand as medics, needs to not exclude or even scare the patient, of course. We need to be aware of how it looks and sounds on 'the other side.' We also need to be aware of how it makes us feel and whether the language reflects actual practice and our values or is outdated and possibly - if even subconsciously - taken literally at some level within trainer or trainee as a spur or challenge, setting an expectation that you have to show you have learnt faster than perhaps you have. In other words, is it dangerous? Words are actions, the philosophers teach us. 'Word acts,' they call them. One of the deep lessons I learnt from facing this potentially life-defining diagnosis is how we rush from task to task and don't have the time for this kind of deep analysis of the meaning of the language we use. Lying in a hospital bed for hours gives that analytical time to you. Or at least to me. And I'm sharing that with you in the hope of it being part of a positive outcome from my experience.

"Yes, I'll be doing it," she said, understanding me exactly. "I'll be showing my colleague how it's done."
"Have you done several?" I asked.
"Yes, I've done plenty," she smiled.
And, at 2:30pm that day, she did the procedure itself very well.

I guess another piece of learning from my experience at this point is that patients who come into hospital are well aware of the pressures on our hospital system; their introduction will often be a long, sometimes distressing wait in A&E. All the evidence is that, because of this knowledge of the pressure on the system, many patients come in with less confidence in our ability to keep them safe and well-looked after in a timely way than a few years ago. Their levels of anxiety are higher. This heightened anxiety, lower trust, creates an extra demand on our time and resources that is rarely commented on, but we need to be aware of, as we all know the impact on outcomes that psychological factors such as stress and anxiety in the patient can have. Trust that is eroded by all the news externally can be pieced back, one by one, with each interaction once the patient comes in. As long as we are all aware of the need. My lumbar puncture doctor gave me the time and the confidence I needed, through how she communicated with me. It was a masterclass in how to reduce stress and anxiety.

As did the brilliant SHO, the Consultants, Registrars, Nurses and (I do need to stress the valuable NHS team includes ancillary staff) the Porters and Healthcare Assistants, Cleaners, and so on, I saw in action also impressed me with this empathy.

The consequence of the lumbar puncture - what it revealed - is something I was less happy with. But that wasn't within her or anyone else's control.

I was told to lay flat in bed while waiting for the results. It was a particularly busy day around me; the next day was a junior doctors' strike.

I don't swear. Well, hardly ever.

At 7.55 p.m., a different Medical Registrar came into the ward and headed straight to me. He introduced himself first.

"I have some bad news," he said, giving me a second to prepare myself. "We found xanthochromia in the lumbar puncture."

Strangely, my hand flew to my head.

"Seriously? F------- Hell!" I heard a voice exclaim. It was me.

Here's an extract from the medical literature for non-medical readers to understand my reaction:

"Xanthochromia is the presence of bilirubin in the cerebrospinal fluid and is sometimes the only sign of an acute subarachnoid haemorrhage."

I did reflect afterwards on my reaction. It was a sudden emotional outburst, uncharacteristic of me. Professor Steve Peters in The Chimp Paradox describes the inner chimp and provides an understanding of how our emotional brains work. It is of course, normal to have these chimp outbursts, particularly in such a stressful moment with the stakes being so high. Exercising my chimp and expressing the emotion was important at that point, followed by the human logical side developing plans for the next steps. I knew it was a likely outcome. Yet responded with a sense of disbelief and an interjection that was unlike me (honest, particularly if my parents are reading this). Such is the power of denial. Again, we know this from when we see patients not wanting to believe bad news, deflecting it if possible, with the familiar response of "I want a second opinion," perhaps in a population with an increased sense of their rights (as it should be) over patients of decades ago. But, to experience that sudden wave of denial, though instantaneous, is instructive. No one is being awkward or unreasonable in how they respond. We (when being medics, not patients) need to read the patient with empathy and interact accordingly. Regardless of the other pressures we are under to communicate and move on. Which is exactly what I experienced; personal communication between healthcare professional and patient at its best, again.

And now it was my turn to practise that level of communicating with care, as I had to pass this unwelcome news on to Sona. Also, to Viren, though, as he's a medic himself, that was more straightforward (though not easy by any means; saying it makes it true, as they say).

I called Viren first. He was surprised but unflustered, as you'd expect. Next, the hardest call to make.

It was 8.30 p.m. or so. Sona was probably putting the kids to bed. I texted to say I was about to call with news. I know her well enough to know this was a kind of - I hoped, gentle - priming for what was about to come.

Then, I followed the training we had for delivering bad news, just as my own doctor had done. I asked if she was sitting down. I said I had some unexpected news, that I knew we were hoping for a negative result, and that I'd be coming home rather than a positive result in the sense of the puncture finding something. Paused a beat to help her absorb. Then told her what the outcome of the lumbar puncture was, a positive finding.

Looking back now, that was the hardest conversation I've ever had - perhaps one of the hardest things I've ever had to do. To deliver such alarming news to the person closest to you in the whole world, whom you would do anything in your power to protect.

Learning point here for any medics reading this: Have you noticed the absolute inversion of the meanings of 'positive' and 'negative' here? We medics call the finding of something a positive result - the LP tested positive. For the recipient of that information, it is not positive, of course; it is entirely negative. Again, words have so much power and as medics we have to think ourselves outside the immediate use of the word - our jargon, if you will - to understand how confusing it can be to report a 'positive' result – a finding – when the non-medical receiver of the wording is likely to be confused by that exactly when they need clarity. They anticipate one of a binary outcome. You appear to be giving them the hoped-for outcome. In microseconds, they compute it as actually the opposite because of the cognitive dissonance between their understanding of 'positive' and the gravity with which you are delivering the news. If you're lucky and they are bright, that is. Can you see the yo-yo bounce in emotions, the massive oscillation on a wave graph that would be produced by us using our jargon version - which flips meaning between leaving our lips and entering the ears and brain of the person we are talking to - as they process the information?

"We're coming now. I'll get the kids looked after," she said.

I told her it was OK, she didn't have to do that; I had scans and other tests to go through now and it was late. But, she insisted. She and Viren drove to Nottingham and the nurses kindly let them stay for half an hour. The need to be together with those who love you and, for them, to be with the person at risk (me, in this case) is compelling when news like this is shared. We all know the research showing the touch of another human - particularly a hand held by a loved one - can actually reduce sense of physical pain, as well as obviously helping psychologically. "You are not going through this alone."

What helped in communicating with Viren and, especially, Sona, was that the incredible team around me had quickly consulted on a plan and had come up with one. The gap between the cliff edge the finding left me at and the rapid construction of a bridge to the other side - the plan - by the medics around me, was phenomenally fast. We all need a way forward, don't we; some certainty of what happens next, if not of ultimate outcome. The brilliant SHO consulting with neurosurgery and keeping me informed as the plan unfolded, then another ward doctor who revisited me several times to give me updates through the evening; this co-ordinated and real-time sharing of information gave me exactly what I needed for my own reassurance and to give me something to share that was positive with Viren and Sona on the phone and when they sat at my bedside. The power of words and of exemplary bedside manner in action.

As an aside, recent research shows that patients are more likely to complain about a doctor who doesn't, in the patient's perception, take the time and care to communicate with evident empathy and clarity. Even taking the outcome into account, a patient is more likely to complain about a poorly communicating doctor when the outcome is good than they are about a doctor they perceive as taking their time and showing empathy, even when the outcome is less good. I'm not mentioning this here as a complaint-avoidance strategy. The avoidance of complaints is merely a beneficial outcome, a symptom if you will, of the underlying sense of trust and confidence the patient forges with a medic and other team members who communicate with empathy, tact and care. Which is what I experienced first hand.

Key points:

1. Trust is central to achieving positive health outcomes in the NHS

2. How we medics communicate - with care and clarity - is as important as what we communicate. And is key to building trust. 'First, do no harm' applies to understanding the impact of the language we use as well as the medical interventions we make. I've reflected, above, on an example: 'positive' and 'negative' having inverse meanings for non-medic versus medics when it comes to test results. For example, if you are a medic, can you reflect on an incident where the use of language may have generated an unintentionally negative outcome for a patient?

3. At its best, as I experienced firsthand, the NHS is full of acts of leadership, at all levels, guided by the common aim of the best interest of the patient.

CHAPTER 3. WHAT THE PATIENT SAW: EXCELLENCE IN ACTION

"We are what we repeatedly do. Therefore excellence is not an act, but a habit." - Will Durant's elegant summation of Aristotle's principle of virtuous actions

When told I had been accepted by neurosurgery, I remember thinking that meant clearly this was serious. I was now a neurosurgery patient. Viren and Sona stayed for about thirty minutes on that second evening spent in hospital. After they left, it was a hard night. I was not sure what the outcome would be, whether I would even survive. The whole night felt long and drawn out. I'm sure the family at home worried too.

I want to stress and give examples here of how my experience in hospital showed me that the NHS team - and its ability to provide exemplary care to patients - is entirely reliant on **and includes** 'ancillary' team members who may at times not be regarded as such. Porters, Cleaners, Catering Managers and Servers, Healthcare Assistants and other 'ancillary' staff are integral, not ancillary, to the care delivered on the wards I was in. I want to give four examples here of excellence observed and experienced, that range from ancillary staff to a surgical team: the porters who ferried me around, a nurse interacting with a trainee, a healthcare assistant feeding a patient, and the theatre team.

The porters

The life of the hospital would grind to a halt without them. As well as moving me around the hospital safely, the porters I encountered were mood-lifters. A nurse came to see me at 6am and told me I'd be heading for a CTA (another, but different, CT scan) later that morning.

Barely thirty minutes later, two cheery porters came in, introduced themselves, carefully transferred me using a pat slide (a patient handling board designed to safely move a patient without straining the back of the person or people moving them) onto a trolley and bantered with me as we headed off to the CT department.

At first, my groggy, sleepless head was resistant to their good humour. It seemed a mismatch with the worried, sleepless, depressed state of mind I was in. But, as we moved through the hospital, I realised their cheeriness was infecting me, lifting me from the worry and preoccupation a little. They were bringing me out of my head, helping me realise this unique and strange experience (for me) was something they did many times each day. I was helpless in their hands. And they handled me with care, expertise and good humour, making me feel safe. Where, at the start of the porter's journey, I had been on my own, inward-focussed, worried, they had teased me out, initiated me into the morning life of the hospital. I wasn't isolated in my own little world of worry. I had companions on this journey. And they were familiar with the territory, experienced travellers who would see me safely through.

Now, whether this cheery raising of my mood was by design or chance, I can't be sure. In an ideal world, the porters would tune themselves to the mood of the patient, you might think: at that hour of the morning, the last thing some patients might want is a dose of cheer. But, what a sombre trip through the corridors that would have been if they'd matched their mood to mine rather than lifting me with their cheeriness.

A quick reference to the medical texts to explain what I was headed for:

"Computed Tomography Angiography (CTA) is a type of medical test that combines a CT scan with an injection of a special dye to produce pictures of blood vessels and tissues in a part of your body. The dye is injected through an intravenous (IV) line started in your arm or hand." **-John Hopkins University**

As the porters took me into the corridor, the Neurosurgical Registrar was there to tell me they had a bed for me in neurosurgery and he would review me in the ward after the CTA. When I went in for the CTA, I felt cold, maybe even nervous, not entirely sure what to expect in terms of findings, even though the procedure itself was one I understood. They gave me an intravenous injection to run dye through my veins. The feeling was peculiar - a flushed feeling as the liquid moved through me. The CTA study was completed quickly and efficiently and I headed to the neurosurgical ward. That morning was non-stop. The neurosurgeon came by, and I told him my recent history - the symptoms and how they'd developed - so that he had it firsthand from me. This was the first step in getting to know and trust the Consultant who would be in charge of overseeing my care. Of which, more later.

On another trip, later in the day, the porters started to accelerate at one point. Now, my worried self, fearing the worse, wondered if they'd been briefed to hurry: why the urgency, I thought. What had I not been told? Daniel Goleman first described the concept of amygdala hijack. This is where the brain reacts immediately and out of proportion to the actual stimulus. I recalled the 6-second rule (it takes six seconds or so for the stimulus of the fight or flight chemicals to calm). Paused. Asking a question would provide me with the answer. But would I like the response? "We're moving fast?" I asked, hesitant to hear the scary response, that getting me there fast was crucial to my survival. "Well, there's an upward slope coming up. We need to build up a bit of speed to get you up it smoothly," said one of the porters.

Like side characters in a Shakespeare play, the good humoured matter of factness of the porters took over the narrative and changed it for me - I was no longer being rushed urgently because if I didn't get there as fast as possible, something terrible might happen to me (the narrative playing in my head). This trip was far more mundane than the drama I had projected onto it. We had a ramp coming, so needed a bit of momentum.

I am reminded of a story about President Kennedy visiting NASA headquarters. As he was shown around Mission Control, asking each member of staff what their role was, he came across a janitor. Not realising the man was there to empty the bins next to the scientists' desks, President Kennedy asked, "And what do you do at NASA?" The janitor answered, "I'm helping to put a man on the moon, sir."

Now, this story may well be apocryphal, but even if it is, the transferable learning is still valid: either this awareness of his role was intrinsic - that he knew by keeping the scientists' work spaces clean and tidy, he was helping them focus their minds on their work, by removing clutter - or a brilliant colleague or supervisor, in an inspired act of leadership, had pointed out to him how vital everyone's role was in achieving the mission, including his, and explained how what the janitor did every day contributed to the goal the whole team existed for, how essential he was to that achievement.

A similar principle applied to my porters, I felt. Their warm, friendly, efficient way of moving me around safely and with care helped tone down in my head the sense that I was in the middle of a personal drama with an uncertain and potentially frightening outcome, and made me appreciate their role in the life of the hospital, transporting patients like me through the veins and arteries of the corridors, if you will, to the vital organs where we needed to be assessed and cured. They were their own little portable centres of excellence, a team of two, whose care I was in as I travelled from ward to scanning centres. Then they handed me over, made sure I was safely in place, wished me a cheery farewell and were off. You cannot underestimate the positive effect on the patient experience of warm, efficient, caring, competent, cheering transactions like those I was on the receiving end of from the hospital porters.

When NHS ancillary members of all kinds are aware of their core mission and role - to help the patient recover and improve - just as that NASA janitor was, just as my porters seemed to be, you get the integrated, holistic levels of care from every encounter that I am bearing witness to in this little book.

My porters also brought to mind a true tale, told to me by a leadership development expert, of a new CEO appointed to a community hospital in the USA. He went undercover on his first day to observe daily life in the hospital at all levels, without the filters that would come from people reporting to or acting in a performative way in front of the CEO. This is an interesting 'back to the floor' (as they call it in leadership development circles) experiment that leaders who are normally based in meetings in board rooms, away from the action and life of an organisation (the shop floor) could benefit from.

In a hospital corridor, the anonymous CEO came across what he thought was a maintenance man with a screwdriver working on the hinges of a pair of push-through doors. He asked the man what he was doing.

"I'm a porter," said the man, continuing to work on the hinges. "Every time I come down this corridor with a patient, in a wheelchair or on a gurney, these doors that are supposed to slide open easily when we make contact with them give us a rude bump. We have to force them. I want my patients to have a smoother ride."

That's exactly the kind of act of leadership at all levels - an initiative taken to make the mission better, to improve the patient experience - that Weber meant in that quote at the top of the previous chapter, over 100 years ago. Does it sound too minor an act of improvement to you to be mentioned here? What if you were a patient with a broken limb or aching head whose mode of transport was jarred by going through those doors, sending small shockwaves up your body and exacerbating your existing discomfort? Or a patient whose muscles were no longer working - such as a patient with Huntington's Disease or some other illness that stops the fine motor movements we all make as part of our autonomous system when lying on a wheeled bed and being moved from place to place, to counter bumps and turns, to keep us stable? Or a patient in a neck brace? In the delivery of healthcare, as we all know - including the porters I encountered and the porter in this story from the USA - there is no such thing as a small thing. A systemic approach – which is the form of leadership mandated by the NHS Leadership Academy as most appropriate and effective in our healthcare system - includes all parts of the system.

A nurse teaching a trainee

From my hospital bed, I guess I was fulfilling the undercover observation role just described in the true anecdote about the American hospital CEO. (Literally undercover, since I was observing from beneath my blanket). One strand of learning that runs through this whole experience for me is about time. I'll go into this more in the next section - how my sense of time passing and how we spend it, at work, at home, when looking forward and backward through my life at any given moment - has been irrevocably changed by the experience I am describing in this book. But for now, I want to focus on one specific element of time - the time medics lack when rushing around the wards from task to task or working through their caseload as GPs with a pre-determined ten minutes per patient, which develops a form of attention deficit, I would argue, in that it limits our awareness of teachable or learnable moments, in the sense of opportunities to step back, observe with that uncluttered mind that is conducive to learning, the action in the hospital or community as it happens.

The 'luxury' to be able to observe in an almost timeless state may be an odd word to use, but the boredom of being in a hospital bed for a length of time, the search for stimulus, for things to learn from, gave me that luxury, mirroring the 'staring out the window' state of mind that none of us have time for today but that the learning experts tell us is the 'tabula rasa' reflective mental state we need to cultivate new insights and learning.

Let me clarify what I mean here: teachable moments and feedback happen all over the NHS all the time. It's how we train on the job. It's how we all improve. The enforced suspension of time, for me, allowed me to observe these teachable moments in action. Ken Blanchard, the leadership guru, said decades ago that a central plank of leadership is to 'catch people doing things right' and then praise and amplify those moments, instilling or reinforcing them in the culture as 'this is the way we do things around here.' Moments of excellence, you might call them. And moments or pockets of excellence are exactly what I observed and experienced and am writing this book partly to share, to expand the audience for the excellence I saw and experienced, if you will.

So, while I was lying in my bed, I observed, for example, a nurse on the other side of the ward from me, showing a student nurse how to set up a paracetamol drip. I marvelled at the way she did it: patiently, expertly. Later that day, she asked the student nurse to set it up herself, supervised of course - the first two of the 'See one, Do one, Teach one' triptych I mentioned earlier as the cycle of learning. Having walked her through the stages, the nurse then reviewed, with the 'how to' manual open between the two of them, mapping each step in the manual onto the real-world experience they were going through. All while both were keeping a focus on the patient, who was relaxed and comfortable throughout. And while feedback on the learning was flowing between the two participants in real-time. We know that we need this feedback to ensure learning has in fact, been passed on, to question and improve, to cement development, and we have various models of post-event feedback that we use in the NHS. But, it was heartening to see 'in action' feedback integrated into the learning in the moment. That was excellence in knowledge transfer right there; a scenario played out hundreds of times a day in each NHS hospital.

A healthcare assistant (HCA) feeding a patient

I watched a healthcare assistant feed a patient in a neighbouring bed. One of the simple fundamentals, you might think: helping people eat, drink, go to the toilet, clean them; all the tasks we entrust HCAs with. Not demanding of a high skillset, surely? But, it's only when we have the time to stop and stare, as I did, that you see how complex this particular 'fundamental' was and how carefully and skilfully it was done. The level of unspoken communication between HCA and patient, the resulting co-ordination of their movement, was a thing of beauty to observe; two humans moving in harmony to a common end, in a complex sequence of signals, responses, movements, that demanded absolute concentration, understanding and trust; that the HCA be completely in tune with the patient.

I watched a manoeuvre that was like the docking of a space shuttle with a space station, for example, in its intricacy: a spoonful of food going into a mouth. Fanciful? Let me explain. First, there's the criticality of the action being undertaken: If a patient has dysphagia (difficulty swallowing), the simple act of eating, an activity meant to nourish and nurture us, could, with one fit of choking, kill us. I watched this spoonful of food being lifted to a mouth, aware acutely of something I'd only been half-aware of previously: that before that food was even chosen, the patient had been assessed for food suitability in a range of four food types, based on the patient's capacity to take in, chew (or not chew) and swallow. The whole meal had been prepared based on one of those four categories. If you include liquids, there are eight levels or categories, ranging from water. Some patients choke on water - the autonomous system doesn't close off the wind pipe with the epiglottis in time, sometimes because the patient's mouth hasn't registered the presence of the water until it's too late (impaired sensitivity or signal transfer within the body) and sometimes because the patient has an impaired ability to control the flow of liquid within the mouth and it hits the back of the mouth too fast. The liquids they are offered in that case need to be one or more levels up from water in terms of their viscosity, and the consequent ability of the mouth to safely move the liquid from front to back of mouth and into the body. That's just the drinks.

With a new level of respect for what the HCA was doing, I watched a spoon of carefully chosen food, of the right consistency for this patient's particular level of swallowing ability, poised in front of the patient, within their line of sight, preparing to dock, so to speak. Awaiting the patient's permission. I watched the HCA watch the patient's eyes, for them to flicker towards the spoon and register it. Timing is everything: present the patient with the next spoon before they have finished processing the food in their mouth and they may feel rushed, start to try and swallow more quickly to prepare for what is coming next. Which is dangerous.

No words were exchanged. Carers and HCAs are taught, or know intuitively, that chatting while eating may be part of the sociability of eating together among well people. But, those who have trouble swallowing need a silent zone in which they and the person with the spoon or feeding cup can operate. There was the tiniest 'go' signal from the patient: the head began to tip back almost imperceptibly, pushing the jaw forward, by a mere millimetre or two, in the direction of the food on the spoon, and the muscles around the mouth started to move in preparation for the lips to open. Synchronicity was triggered as if the autonomous nervous system now extended between the two people, co-ordinating their movements: the spoon started to move, gently, just as the head moved, reaching the lips and resting on the lower one for a beat, allowing the patient to register that it was there through the sensation on their lower lip. The HCA didn't push the spoon: the patient enveloped it with their mouth. The HCA smoothly performed a gentle reverse scooping movement with the spoon, extricating it from the mouth in an upward curved movement (preventing spillage) and then taking it out of the patient's line of sight. Most feeders - say if you're feeding a baby - would follow the spoon with their eyes back down to the bowl to refill it. This HCA watched the patient, not the spoon. To make sure there was no discomfort provoked by the food added to the mouth; that it wasn't too much, that the mouth, tongue and throat movements were co-ordinating as they should. That there was no hint of incipient choking prompted by the new input of food. And that the patient was enjoying their food. You can tell. There's a kind of unspoken, unsounded 'mmmm' you can see on the face.

Even this spoon wasn't an ordinary spoon. People with dysphagia, particularly if they have an illness that makes it difficult for them to co-ordinate mouth movements smoothly, may jerk towards a metal spoon, the impulse of hunger coupled with lack of muscle control can lead to damage to the inside of the mouth with a metal spoon. There is a range of soft plastic spoons matched with the different consistencies of food and different capacities of different patients. All of these half-forgotten, buried facts that we pay no attention to welled up in my head to explain the nourishing two-step slow dance of trust, empathy and nurturing that was going on with this one spoonful of food.

The catering managers and servers who brought the food around to people like me were catering - literally - to a phenomenal range of needs, from my simple ones to the complex needs I have just described, and doing so deftly, with kindness and a smile and impeccable timing. Critical tasks performed brilliantly and vital to the patient's health and wellbeing. So, you see what I mean about my raised level of awareness, through observation, of how there is one NHS team delivering care, and it encompasses experts whom some might see as ancillary workers, on the edge of the patient experience and incidental to the health and wellbeing of the patient. Not so. I saw and experienced their centrality to the one team, to the delivery of excellent care, for myself.

A vision appears

I want to remind us all of the emotional lift of the familiar when we are in the unfamiliar surroundings of a hospital ward. After the CTA experience mentioned above, and the bedside chat from the consultant, I saw, on the ward, trotting towards me, a familiar figure, a blast from the past, you might say. It was one of my old friends I had studied with at university. The strangeness of this was akin to coming across an oasis in the desert, perhaps. No disrespect to the wonderful people around me who had been looking after me - they were exemplary. But, they were unfamiliar, part of the new world of 'Amit the patient' who had been struck down. Here was a reminder that my life before then was real and still ongoing. I was not in completely unknown territory. Here was someone who knew me from before, providing a thread of continuity from that life into this hospital experience. I grasped at it delightedly. I can't tell you how reassuring and what a lift it gives you when someone familiar, from your past life, so to speak, steps into focus in the unfamiliar world into which you have been plunged. The incongruity of it - the unexpectedness of this old friend trotting towards me - brought a rush of warmth and gave me a lift. He instantly put my mind at ease, was calm and reassuring. I asked about the next steps, and he suggested we wait for the consultant ward round rather than conject what might happen.

The ward round did come soon after. The CTA was reported normal. The plan, said the consultant, was to refer me to an interventional radiologist, himself a consultant. In the meantime, Viren and Sona were downstairs already that morning waiting for updates. When the interventional radiologist came, he had with him two junior doctors. Bearing in mind the junior doctor strike was on that day, I was impressed.

The consultant radiologist, who would be in charge of the theatre team, inspired trust immediately. He was well-spoken, both eloquent and empathetic. He told me that the gold standard test was the DSA.

DSA? I'll let a quote from the medical literature explain:

"Digital subtraction angiography (DSA) is a diagnostic procedure to view the inner surface of blood vessels (also known as lumen). It can be used to view arteries, veins and heart chambers. DSA is a fluoroscopic technique (a technique that captures continuous images) that uses complex, computerised X-ray machines."

He explained what it would involve and why it was necessary, but that it carried with it a 1 in 100 risk of an ischaemic stroke.

From the nature and tone of the conversation so far - from what he told me to how he told me, from the way he listened and responded - I already trusted him implicitly. I looked him in the eye and said, "Do what you need to do; I've got full faith in you."

He had completed a consent form, assuming my response, which I signed promptly as he wanted to take me downstairs ASAP to theatre. One more impressive thing about this interaction was that, before I had the chance to raise it, he asked who else I needed him to speak to. The awareness of me as not just an individual patient, but someone with loved ones, and that he needed to include them in this conversation, with my guidance and permission, was impressive. I obviously wanted my wife and brother to be aware, particularly of the stroke risk, and we called Sona and Viren up from downstairs so he could talk with them.

This stroke, induced by the procedure, has consequences for the family too, of course, so he explained the risk, just as he had done with me, and asked if they were prepared to accept the risk. The alternative was obviously more dangerous - leaving what was going on in my brain as a mystery that could do me more harm unless investigated properly with the DSA.

As the consultant talked about the risk, I remember Sona staring at me with renewed concern. She didn't say anything but what I read in her eyes was, "The stakes are increasing here Amit!"

While Sona and I communed silently, Viren was asking questions and seeking reassurance from the consultant. In these conversations, there is what is actually being said and the subtext. The subtext from Viren to the consultant was, "Look after my brother. Reassure me that you will all look after my brother. He is much-loved."

The trust the consultant inspired in us at that moment was immeasurable, worth all the money in the world.

Then they went, and I waited. But, not for long, as my friendly neighbourhood porters turned up again quite quickly, telling me MRI had called and wanted me down there for an MRI scan now.

Such is your level of anxiety when you are a patient waiting for a procedure, that I found myself thinking, "Why now all of a sudden? What's wrong with me that I have to be rushed to MRI?" On reflection, no matter how clear the planning, no matter how well communicated with the patient this is, there will be the issue of availability of a window opening up, a slot becoming available. That was the reality. Stopping the anxiety in your head imposing a different, more alarming reality, is an ongoing piece of work in a hospital stay. What doesn't help is that, on this occasion, the pain in my head and the stiffness in my neck had moved up another notch and were becoming unbearable. We all know how disorienting pain is. And how alarming it can be when it continues to escalate.

If you've experienced an MRI scan, you'll know it's loud - as if your head is being put in a piece of industrial machinery. You have ear protection and obviously have to keep as still as possible, all the while wondering what the massive magnets revolving around your head are revealing as you lie as still as you can on the bed of the scanner. The team doing the investigation are behind glass, as only you can be in the room. It's a lonely place to be. And you are there for quite a while, the magnets making odd bursts of sound, differing patterns of noises that, if you let your imagination run, could leave you feeling you are in an alien spacecraft. You find yourself trying to interpret the different pulses, mark the change of patterns from one to the other, try and imagine what they signify.

I was in there for over an hour. They had to pause after 40 minutes to reposition. At which point, the radiologist made a decision to give me contrast (injecting a contrast dye) as they needed a clearer view. This raised my anxiety levels: What had they found? Why did we now need contrast?

The radiographer came and spoke to me, which was reassuring, then injected the contrast, producing a warm feeling that ran up my arm.

The scan resumed for another twenty minutes or so, after which they now told me they wanted to take me straight to theatre. I had assumed I would return to the ward to decompress and recover from the thumping, whining and pulsing of the MRI machine, which can leave you feeling wrung out. It's not easy keeping still for that long, particularly when in pain. So, the unexpected news that I would be going straight to theatre raised the anxiety levels still further.

That journey was hard with the porters. I couldn't help thinking "What have they found?" My neck pain was really bad. This was the journey mentioned earlier where they had to run at one point, accelerating to negotiate the approaching upward slant in the corridor, with a part of me feeling this need for speed was in fact a consequence of something terrible about to happen to me, so they were rushing to head it off.

The theatre team

When I was taken into theatre for the DSA procedure, the stakes were raised, as Sona's meaningful, wordless gaze had acknowledged. It's known as the gold standard test for tracking down exactly what is happening in your head and where. The stakes were raised because DSA is more invasive than the CTA and MRI scans. And that comes with a risk. As the consultant had explained, there was a 1 in 100 chance of me, the patient, experiencing a stroke because of it. It's on a different level, an interventionist level, to the earlier scans, and that's why I was in theatre, surrounded by a team led by an interventional radiologist. And this is, again, where I observed excellence in action that I want to share.

During my long night on the ward, I had scribbled in a notebook, writing down what I had observed so far, examples of NHS values being lived every day. I've shared a few with you here already. In the long, sleepless night, there was a sense of calm, of being well looked after, helped by looking out through my window at the peaceful night sky and the lights of the city. In the illuminating cone from my bed reading light, I wrote down what I had observed and experienced so far, a series of words I had seen in action: 'negotiations, development of trust, respect, autonomy, listening, defined roles and responsibilities enhancing the effectiveness of teamwork.' I wrote down 'authenticity.' I wrote down 'empowering the teams, teaching, training, learning and feedback.' These were core values being played out with skill that I observed during my stay in hospital, none more so than in this most intense episode of my stay, my time in surgery.

I've tried to live my life with those principles and values and achieve and develop those levels of leadership when I practise medicine. Shared principles and values provide, underpin and inform the culture, the 'way we do things around here' in an organisation. I had become acutely aware that I had moved from practitioner to observer of these values in action. That actually what I was doing now, as well as personally experiencing excellent healthcare as a result of those lived values, was the meta role of bearing witness to them. I had learnt these values and principles myself, did everything in my power to live them at work, put them into practice, and now I was witnessing and providing feedback (via this book).

There was a journey here - one that I am still on - that I travelled through alongside my patient journey, that I am still travelling through now, which is a reflection on leadership. To jump ahead a little, the journey of leadership has been described as ultimately making yourself unnecessary. It was the American campaigner Ralph Nader who identified that "The function of leadership is to produce more leaders, not followers." Ultimately, it is to make yourself replaceable as a do-er. Perhaps observing, recording, witnessing and teaching is the ultimate in disseminating leadership. After you have helped develop as many leaders as possible within the system by example, by doing, of course. "Leadership is example, that's all it is," a great clinician said once, and I am sharing powerful examples here, as that sharing can be a catalyst for the mimetic nature of leadership - how it spreads throughout an organisation, by example, from person to person. As long as we keep that 'learning eye' open and scanning, as long as we consciously look for examples of excellence while we are rushing through the tasks of the day, not allowing the landscape to become a blur, but being able to home in on the detail, as that's where excellence in healthcare lives.

Warren Bennis, who was known as 'the father of leadership theory', more or less inventing it as an academic discipline, has described the stages of leadership development as starting out as an inward analysis - focus on developing the self - the skills I need, the type of person I need to be and so on. And then, when you really mature as a leader, everything is about others. It's about observing them, helping them, embedding leadership in the system, observing leadership in the system, calling out by example where it's working best. Which is what I hope I am achieving here. That set of values in action that I scribbled into my notebook is definitely what I observed and experienced in this crucible moment on my patient journey, in the operating theatre. This was the pinnacle of those values in action on my patient journey, in fact.

As I've described, I was called down to theatre - of course, the availability heuristic was at work here again. There was I thinking "Why am I being rushed there now?" Because the team had gathered, the theatre was booked and they were ready for me is the answer. It was my time. Anxiety of course increases as you enter theatre. But, what I observed had the opposite effect, actually filling me with awe and a sense of being in the middle of, the subject of, a performance of team excellence that was as inspiring as if I were in a different kind of theatre watching the most uplifting, jaw-dropping performance of experts at the pinnacle of their field - If you're a ballet afficionado, say, and can imagine being transported by seeing the most iconic ballerina of her generation, performing with a troupe of unrivalled skill and beauty, just for you, an audience of one.

What I observed was teamwork like an oiled machine. I registered the nurse doing my obs (observations), the scrub nurse recapping my history to focus the team on why we were here, how we had got here, and what the consequent task in hand was. I observed the Consultant and juniors choosing and arranging the equipment quietly, getting everything ready and to hand.

As I entered the main theatre, I was told about the next steps. The Consultant told me he was about to talk to the juniors who would be observing the DSA, almost as if asking permission to move on to that step. "That's fine," I said. Listening in would give me a chance to remind myself of cranial arterial anatomy!

Where this kind of skilled inclusion of the patient in the conversation can help with vulnerability, when it came to dignity, there wasn't much that could be done to alter the fact that I was the one who had to remove what little clothes I had on. They asked me if I could lower my underwear. I responded, "I've left my dignity at the door. Just do whatever you need to do."

In that moment, where having to remove what clothing you have left is peeling away a final layer of protection - if you've ever had those dreams of being naked and exposed while surrounded by strangers in a public place, you know what a fear that is in our minds - you could see the professionalism coming through from the team, in the depths of, from my perception, my own vulnerability.

It is important to acknowledge vulnerability. What is it? I looked it up later. It's defined as "The state of being exposed to the possibility of being attacked or harmed either physically or emotionally" (OED). I felt vulnerable yet the environment was cultivated such that there was trust, collaboration, conversations in order to reach a successful outcome, reducing the risks, ameliorating my sense of vulnerability and the anxiety that sense of powerlessness can give rise to.

Empathy in recognising vulnerability allows us to develop a deeper understanding in defining true leadership. Recognising the challenge or emotional struggle the patient may be going through - 'seeing' the sense of weakness - allows the team to cultivate a position altogether to reassure the patient for a successful outcome.

After a local anaesthetic, a catheter inserted into my groin allowed them to navigate up the arteries to the chest, through the neck and into the brain. The consultant squirted the contrast with the radiographer taking x-rays at various points to identify the location. They worked sequentially - squirt then take the x-ray - repeatedly, and almost without words, a low murmur between them as they worked together. It felt to me as if 'The Force' were at work between them, guiding both their actions. The consultant continued talking to the team as the X-rays were taken. Once the dye reached the brain, the important stuff started. Where was the bleed?

The consultant told me I would feel an odd sensation at various stages and I did. The contrast dye, which helps the blood vessels show up, produced a flushing sensation through certain parts of my head as it moved across. There was a metallic taste in my mouth and a kind of 'rippling' phenomenon or sensation, which I thought felt decidedly odd. It only lasted a few minutes.

At the end of the procedure, I was taken to recovery where I was told everything looks reassuring. Crucially, no specific bleed was obvious but they would need to look at the images more closely while I recovered.

After an hour in recovery, I was moved back to my ward. Sona and Viren came up to keep me company. Later that evening, at about 7 p.m., my neurosurgery consultant arrived to report the findings to us. He said it's likely the bleed is venous or capillary in origin - a *perimesencephalic* SAH - rather than arterial and that observation over the next few days would be crucial. Now, this was a desired outcome - a better prognosis than if it had been an arterial bleed. So, there was some relief in the reported findings there. But, there was and still is a sense of mystery. We know it wasn't an aneurysm bleed. If it had been, that could have been dealt with using clips and coils to seal it off, and the story is over. The culprit is found and made harmless, as with all good detective stories. Unfortunately, we often have to learn to live with the grey of uncertainty rather than the black or white of a clear finding. And this remains the case for me. We didn't find the exact cause, didn't pinpoint the scene of the crime, to continue that analogy of detection. This is, it's true, harder to deal with: shades of grey make it less certain when I can go back to exercising, for example. But, uncertainty is a challenge we all have to live with. The difference is simply of degree. The plan was that if everything was stable I would be discharged after the weekend. With follow up imaging in 6-8 weeks to check all was well. And that's how I see the way forward now, as I write this, over three months after the event. The aim was to get to six weeks. That milestone was successfully passed. Now I am past the three month marker, I am looking to phase myself back into work in this 3-6 month period of recovery. Each marker passed is a success.

He also arranged a neurological review to explore further the cause of the SAH. So far, we haven't gotten to the bottom of it, and we may never do so.

It was during my weekend on the ward while being monitored that I recorded some of the moments of excellence I shared earlier in this chapter. Time went so slow; there was a constant searching for stimuli among the boredom of bed rest and observation that at least I could act as an observer, looking out for moments of excellence to record and share here.

At the same time, the pain hadn't gone away. As well as managing the headache, the painful and stiff neck, there was a developing lower back pain to be managed. I wasn't fully healed yet, obviously, and the consequences of the event in my head were still working their way through, so we needed time to see how this would unfold.

Key points

This chapter is mainly about the excellence in action I observed in ancillary staff and in theatre, the crucible of my visit. What made the NHS colleagues I observed in action such an exceptional team? I observed in action these ten essential attributes, which sum up the learning from my experiences and observations detailed in this chapter:

1 Trust
2 Assigned roles/responsibility
3 Verifying checks (double/triple)
4 Communicating effectively
5 Empathy and compassion
6 Positive mindset
7 Learning culture
8 Empowering
9 Receptivity to feedback
10 Inspiration

CHAPTER 4. ABOUT TIME

"Growth comes from chaos, not order."
Rakesh Jhunjhunwala

The Amit who came home had changed from the Amit who went into hospital. The chaos of being knocked out of the timeline of my life - as I saw it - and into a life-threatening situation had stimulated a form of growth as a person that couldn't have come, I believe, if life had carried on as normal before.

The Thunderclap inside my head brought fear, pain, worry for everyone and the risk of my death. But it also brought a transformational change to me, to how I perceive myself, my past and future, the people around me whom I love, and my purpose in life. Time seemed and still seems different. Maybe being thrown out of the timeline you thought you were in does that.

I became aware of this while still in hospital, in that long second night, when I was awake and pondering.

They say that when you die, your life flashes before your eyes. I'm glad to say I can neither confirm nor deny that. But, what I can report is what happened to me when I was visited by a life-threatening event, one that made me consider my own mortality. When you consider your own death, it inevitably, it turns out, makes you look at your life.

When I lay awake at night in that hospital bed, staring out the window, making notes in my little book, having been told I was in the aftermath of - and maybe still in the middle of - a life-threatening event, memories of that life were playing across my mind like scenes in a film. And they weren't the scenes you might expect. What was important to me seemed to have shifted, the foundations moved and reset themselves. Or things I had considered as marginal, the small things, were reasserting themselves as the big things. Here are 12 things that popped into my head, that I scribbled down that night.

Twelve life memories

1. One of my early memories is when my dad would give us "piggyback" rides from one side of the room to the other. A small thing that taught me, I now realise, what unconditional love is. He could have thought he had better things to do for us than that - he was a driven man in the amount of work hours he put in for his family, as I have said. But, that time spent playing with us is what I remember.

2. Dad teaching my brother and me how to ride our BMX bikes. First with the stabilisers and then getting our confidence up to ride without. We would practise down the street, using the kerb as a support should we need it

sometimes. It gave us confidence and trust that we could learn how to do something scary.

3. Mum would take us to the city centre, to the famous Leicester Market. I remember lots of people shouting and trying to sell their fresh fruit and vegetables. We learnt about negotiation, transactions. Whilst this was fun, carrying all the bags back home on the bus was always a challenge! I also recall Mum getting clothes for Dad from a shop called C&A and the frustration my dad would share when she had overspent, in his eyes. She only ever overspent on him (never herself) because he needed a shirt or something. Despite his protests, he would always love wearing the clothes. I learnt how easy it is to spend hard-earnt money, and to be wary of that. But, also how self-denial sometimes needs to be overcome by another's love (Mum bought for Dad what he wouldn't buy for himself).

4. Another memory is my brother always coming to support me when I was playing a football match without fail. When I was 14 and he was 12 he would train me at home and encourage me to improve. He'd make me run around him while he stood still in the middle. He is my massive supporter and has always been a rock. Sacrificing your time to support others is no sacrifice at all. It is, once again, an act of love and nurturing.

5. Winning Student of the Year in year 11 in a regional competition after being nominated and going through a rigorous interview! My folks were pleased, though we were running late for the presentation ceremony. But that's my parents: always working hard. Every parents' evening, we

never made it on time. Because they'd be working so late, and sometimes would have to borrow a car to get there on time, as we didn't have one. The teachers would sometimes have to wait for them. The look in their eyes, though, told us they were proud of Viren and me. It helped that our reports weren't bad.

6. Becoming a doctor and being able to help others and give to society. See point 12, below, for how this links to my Grandma.

7. Spending a big chunk of my first year's income on a BMW. My dad often says a car gets you from a to b but when he and my brother went to see it, he even said, "If you like it, just get it, Amit". He was almost giving me permission, saying you've put the work in, enjoy it.

8. Part 2 of the BMW story. When dating my to-be wife, on the second date I picked her up from a London station in my car. As she climbed in, she said, "Nice ride." That car was made for that moment.

9. Our wedding day in Kenya and spending time with Sona's parents, getting to know them and her family better. Indeed a very special moment. Sona often says that marriage is also about bringing families together, and I am very fortunate to have spent quality time with Sona's parents (Nilesh and Bharti) but also sister and brother-in-law (Shital and Alpesh).

10. Our honeymoon in the Maldives: the sunsets with Sona are locked in my mind. We have also journeyed across the globe, visiting Cambodia, Vietnam, Mexico, Mauritius,

Italy, France, Thailand to name a few. Creating memories that matter.

11. Rian and then Siya being born. With Rian it was indescribable, the best feeling ever, particularly as he was the first. I just loved his smile. With Siya that, too, was a magical moment. She was a January baby and I recall how we had the BMW ready and packed. But it snowed. We had just got a Land Rover, which we had no intention of taking, but had no choice but to swap cars at 1am at night, moving everything over to the four-wheel drive car, which was safer in the snow. Now, we always say, "Siya wanted to come in style!"

12. My Mum's and my Grandma's amazing cooking. Never to be forgotten. Grandma love gives you a licence and autonomy, a different approach to generational love than the direct guidance of a parent. They give you opportunities to develop in more ways than you can imagine. The intensity of that love, for me, is remembered in the food. My grandma made these amazing Indian pancakes called pudla. She'd make the batter, mixed in with fresh coriander. And then she shallow fries it in the pan - I'm seeing it now, it's that vivid - flips it over. Oh and the softness inside but also the crispiness on the outside, eaten with a spice - imagine sweet mango that's pickled; heavenly! The importance of intense moments, symbolising care and love like this, is that they live with us, travelling down through the years. I had conversations with my Grandma where I remember telling her I'd like to be able to care for people. She made it clear she'd always wanted a doctor in the

family to do just that. And Viren and I became medics. She never got to see us graduate in becoming doctors. But, she helped inspire it. Partly through the love put into those pudlas and digested by us, I suspect. Dreams drive us. Without them, we are but shadows.

There were other memories, of course, that were dear to me: friends, mentors flitted across my mind, whom I was so happy to have known. But, piggy backs? Shopping in Leicester market? Not what you might expect to come front of mind as significant, memorable life events.

Purpose: what are you for?

On that long night in the hospital, I also found myself wondering what I was for. What's my purpose?

Like everyone else, I raced through each day, ticking off tasks done, letting moments fly past. In the race rather than in the moment. On a Saturday, the kids might say, "Let's go out to play." And we do. But, a thought pops into my head, I pull my phone out and start making notes for the Partners' Meeting on Monday. My mind is half there instead of in the moment with my children.

A brush with mortality brings a re-evaluation of purpose - what are we here for? Aristotle's theory of purpose focussed on living life as a series of virtuous acts that equate to *eudaimonia* - loosely defined as 'happiness' but more literally as 'well being' - living life well in and for itself rather than 'happiness' being an outcome, something to be 'pursued', as the US constitution puts it. I pondered purpose, noted how it gives you direction, intentions and objectives. When you are successful, it gives you rewards. But how do I define success and what's important? Is it based on financial reward, position, a sense of winning, of recognition? My brain was free-forming, examining fundamentals I had not really looked at in this kind of granular detail before, examining myself and what I did forensically.

We assume action brings reward; the point of the action becomes the reward. Recognition is often the form the reward comes in. Now, I've always been aware of ego, wary of it as a reason for doing things. Isn't the reward system, though dressed up as 'purpose', pandering to my ego? As you can see, I was coming up with questions about how we live today that were pointing me back at the Aristotlean idea of happiness as living within what we do, not as a reward *for* what we do.

But, I did make some headway, a deeper level of self-analysis than the cursory glance we give ourselves when we think we are analysing our motivations, why we do what we do. That jumped me back in time, leapfrogging Aristotle's teacher Plato, to *his* teacher Socrates, and his fundamental insight that **the unexamined life is not worth living**. My enforced inactivity, being withdrawn from the 'rat race' so to speak, and given time to observe and reflect, was giving me the space to do a whole lot of examining.

I also pondered a more recent insight, John F Kennedy's quote that "Effort and courage are not enough without purpose and direction." Yes, my purpose is to serve, to give. But, after this particular life event, do I resolve to give more?

To give differently? When you re-evaluate what is important in your life, your mind goes to the need for balance. Balancing work with the home, the family, personal life takes on a new sense of urgency.

The actions that we are often rewarded for, recognised for, that deliver achievements to us, are in fact the prize. You are what you do. Reward doesn't lie in the achievement or coming out of the action. The action is in and of itself sufficient. Let me explain that better: someone may be recognised for charity services for homeless people. But this 'honouring' is not the actual reward. The reward is the action that puts a roof over the heads of vulnerable people. The person who spontaneously sits down on the pavement with a homeless person and, unobserved, keeps them company, talks with them, shows them warmth and care ... the act itself, if it helps that person, is its own reward. It doesn't need acknowledging.

The small acts of kindness in our lives are the big things, are they not? So, if reward is **in** actions, how do you get everyone to live that way? How, in, say, the workplace, do you create alignment of the vision, whatever that might be, with action? We will all be familiar with these terms: fairness, equity, consistency, teamwork, respect, negotiation, compassion, positive compromise - these are key attributes to allow one to achieve rewards in actions.

That's the kind of fundamental reassessment of purpose, of self-questioning, I was and am still going through.

I'll share here a few insights from the great Indian philosopher Tagore that have helped me focus on some of these reassessments of my life and purpose:

"I slept and dreamt that life was joy. I awoke and saw that life was
service. I acted and behold, service was joy."

So, someone clearly got there before me in spotting the false idea that reward (joy) is separate from and comes out of beneficial actions (service). The service itself is the point, the purpose, the joy.

"It is very simple to be happy, but it is very difficult to be simple."

Those simple memories I listed above are and were a source of happiness. Yet it is difficult, among the complexity of the demands on us at work, in a complex system like healthcare, to keep sight of the simple things that matter, doing the right thing in work and life, small kindnesses.

"We come nearest to the great when we are great in humility."

Now, that one speaks to me as it is anti-ego and I feel ego is the enemy of service, something to be feared, as I said. In the last chapter, I mentioned Warren Bennis's insight that in leadership you start out focused on yourself, honing your skills, wanting to improve your impact as a leader, learning how to do it, and then develop into mature leadership, which has a selflessness about it, being all about developing others.

I find this really useful in terms of reconsidering my purpose. Because where I used to sit, the leadership positions I occupied are currently an empty chair, while I am off work recuperating. Did I do enough to develop the people around me, who will be filling that chair, so that it doesn't matter in effect that I'm not there? Sounds odd, doesn't it, "Doesn't matter if I'm not there." But if you look ahead, think of time differently, think of legacy and empowering and equipping people to sit in your chair, to do a better job of it than you are doing, then that's a level of leadership that ultimately aims for your own redundancy. You can't get more ego-lite than that.

And why wait until you are gone? As Lao Tse is supposed to have said,

"The great leader is he (or she, of course) of whom the people say, 'We did it ourselves.'"

This takes us back to fostering and nurturing and enabling acts of leadership within the system. Perhaps the best we can be is an authentic example, whether we can be seen or not. The acts of service we perform aren't performative. They are just what we do and who we are. These acts become mimetic - other people around you unconsciously act more in alignment with the values you exemplify; that's how culture spreads and is reinforced. And you do the same when you spot values being lived in small acts by your colleagues, that amplifies your own commitment to the cause, so to speak. We inspire each other, in other words. Of course, it's the same even when there is no example to give, when no-one is there to see: "Who are you when no-one's looking?" is a question some leadership development people use to challenge leaders. Exactly the same as when people **are** looking is the ideal answer, of course. Authenticity is one of the words I wrote down in my hospital bed at night, as part of the list of qualities and values I had seen in action and experienced myself from the NHS colleagues around me. Undercover, sometimes, remember, when they didn't know they were being observed.

Love is the thing

I did something strange to my dad, that I'd never done before, when I got home from hospital. He came upstairs to the bedroom to see me. I said, "Dad, you know, I love you, right?" He's not a man who says, I love you. He stood there, quiet. Then I said, "Dad, you're not going to say it back to me? Really?" I made him say it back to me.

Yes, I know he loves me. But, at this inflexion point in my life, I need to make sure the people I love know I love them, that it is out in the open, surfaced, not just taken for granted. I wanted him to actually say it and not be that quiet male figure that I've always been used to in my life, who doesn't talk about such thing. He doesn't break down or appear emotional. He looks at everything and tackles it head-on. He's a very intelligent man, who is also a man of few words. He'd look at my maths books with me, for example, when I was a kid. I was good at maths, but occasionally would make an avoidable error, a lapse of concentration. My teacher would write in the margin SS - Silly Slip - for those moments. Dad would come in on these and ask, "What happened there?" Always looking to improve, focusing on the bit that needed fixing. Now, that can come across as a disciplinarian, but it's how he focused me on not being smug about the majority I'd got right and think about avoiding Silly Slips, areas to improve. My dad is very much a giver. He will give if you need, a man of action, not words.

I had real pain in my legs and was unable to walk when I got back. We don't have a recliner chair among our furniture at home. So, Dad and Viren got hold of one and brought it to my house, put a thick duvet on it for comfort so I could sit in the living room, reclining when needed, as part of my recovery. See what I mean: acts of love, not words. I made him say it anyway.

And I showered my mum with kisses, which I hadn't done since I was much younger. My mum is another pillar of strength. I view her as the goddess of strength - relentless, focussed and dedicated. She would sit with me in the afternoons during my recovery and we would chat, reconnect; something I missed in my life.

Sona, Viren and Anisha are essential to my recovery as, of course, are my wonderful children. My healing and recovery are a family effort and everything - from Viren's sharing of his analytical brain and support in the hospital to Anisha caring for the children to allow Sona to be with me - was noticed with an enormous sense of appreciation. But, talking of small acts of kindness, acts of love and, in the last chapter, of vulnerability and getting used to accepting care, not just seeing myself as the healthcare giver, I must mention Sona's mother and father, my in-laws.

They were on holiday in Canada when I fell ill and was admitted to hospital. They cut short their vacation to come back and support myself and Sona. They came to visit me in the hospital. Then, when I got back from the hospital, and they became aware of the problem with my lower back pain and leg issues - that I was unable to walk and in a lot of pain. The doctor prescribed oramorph (morphine) and paracetamol for the pain , but I tend not to take painkillers if I can avoid it. Sona's mother began to give me massages to help me get better and ease the pain. I said thank you, no, at first, not wanting to be a bother - possibly that habit of a health caregiver struggling to accept being a recipient - but I then accepted. Acceptance is something we all need to learn, sometimes; to accept what for others is an act of family love. My legs got stronger, the pain receded, and I could walk downstairs again. What can I say? Talk about cradled with the love of my family when I need it most.

Conclusion. So, what next?

The quote at the beginning of this chapter says, "Growth comes from chaos, not order". This is perhaps the most surprising deep learning for me that arose from this episode in my life. In chaos, you don't know what is happening next. I didn't know what was going on in my own head. There was this state of not knowing - something we usually fear and feel uncomfortable within - and there was chaos not only around me, physically, but also mentally in my own headspace. But in that journey and that process, I feel I have grown as an individual and as a person, received insights from that period of chaos that I otherwise would not have done. I would have just carried on doing what I was doing and thinking, and what I thought was reflection and learning, I now see as largely superficial. The time and space I've had during and following these events allowed for a deeper reflection. It was a revelation to me that growth comes from chaos. And a massive positive that emerges from what could otherwise be seen as a wholly negative experience.

A Chilean philosopher and computer scientist, Fernando Flores, when sitting in a prison cell where he had been cast by a political opponent for two years, came up with a taxonomy for what we know and what we don't know and how we can progress and transform - both ourselves and our organisations.

He said there are three realms: *what you know you know,* which is the smallest and most self-limiting; *what you know you don't know,* which is the learning path we try and follow, as clinicians, and is codified and laid out before us in training, teaching and courses, as well as referring patients to other experts who have deep knowledge of an area where we know we don't have that depth of expertise. The third area of awareness and knowledge of the world is the least visited by any of us; *what you don't know you don't know,* which is the richest area of all in terms of growth and awareness and yet one which many of us never get to visit. In fact, we shun it because it is not a comfortable place to be. It is a place of chaos, with (unlike the second category of awareness) no clear path forward. Yet, says Flores, "To live in this realm is to notice opportunities that we're normally too blind to see. Transformational opportunities." And transformational truths, because we see without bias.

I feel that's where I've been - a period of chaos that revealed truths about: what I hold dear; about the passage of time and how we need to live and operate within it, relishing moments of love, spotting and grasping teachable moments at work; about purpose - what I am here for, what I need to be for my family and community, the people I serve; how values are lived within the NHS I love and work in, and how those values will sustain the NHS through its own period of (to some extent) chaos, as the principles underlying our healthcare system and the people working within it are stressed as never before. The excellence of care I received within a stressed system is evidence of what lived principles in action can achieve. I will strive to help share that learning and to further it through my own leadership and developing the leadership of others, championing authenticity and lived values. This book, sharing my experiences of NHS healthcare, is part of that commitment to dissemination.

What this period of unstructured learning reminds me of, in fact, is the elective year I took, travelling the world and studying other health systems. While having a wildly exciting time, of course. I was only 22 after all. That was a period of unstructured learning, rather than staying in my known learning lane, if you will. And the learning that comes out of that, the growth that comes out of opening your mind to the outside world, the world of the unknown, is that you don't know what you're going to learn in unknown places until you go there. Exactly as Flores said. You need almost an active faith that the learning out there is as valuable as the prescribed learning in your courses.

I have emerged from this intense period of learning determined to be a better version of myself. But, I hope you don't feel the past few paragraphs sound grandiose. I'd like to emphasise the opposite - the importance of moments, of small things, daily interactions and relationships. Let me end with a suitably small example:

Rian is five and a half. He asked me the other day, almost randomly in a conversation, "Dad, how do I get a litter picker?" First bit of learning there, I guess, is that if you don't make time with your kids and others for these random things to emerge from conversation, they never will. The importance of being present in the moment. Make time (note to self) for more of them. Also, as an aside, way back at the beginning of this book, you may recall when I had to phone Sona in the middle of a workday to come take me to the hospital, I mentioned that she would wonder why I was ringing, that something must be wrong, because I never do that: we never have lunch together in the working week. That's something else small that needs changing.

I asked Rian why he needed a litter picker. He had just got a Blue Peter badge and had his eye on a Green badge the TV programme has introduced for Green activities in the community. We'd helped him write off for the original badge, and he wanted to do it again for the new, Green badge. He wanted to get a badge for his sister Siya, too, so this wasn't just a selfish exercise in accumulation. And he'd decided on litter collection as he thought this was important for the environment. Pretty sound thinking for a five-year-old. We discussed it, and he agreed that the point of the litter picker was to carry on living out, in daily small ways, the values the Green badge represented. That was the discussion we had. He agreed to pick up litter as a habit, regularly, for a year before writing off for the Green badge. That distinction I mentioned earlier between action and reward, that the action or service is the reward itself? My son knows that. I did, though, also say to enjoy the first badge. It's special. You see, everything in life has a time, purpose, worth and reward, depending upon your perspective.

My learning from chaos has been quite the opposite of grandiose; it is rather about the cumulative importance of small things. Life is a series of moments. Transformational growth lies in a multitude of constant acts of kindness, thoughtfulness and learning, enacted in moments, as I've tried to illustrate when outlining the moments of excellence within my hospital stay and the moments of importance in my life as I reflect back on it with renewed clarity. We change ourselves, each other, our healthcare system, and the world one small interaction at a time.

Printed in Great Britain
by Amazon

44749737R00050